Primer on Prostate Cancer

Primer on Prostate Cancer

Nicholas James
Professor of Clinical Oncology
Queen Elizabeth Hospital Birmingham
Birmingham, UK

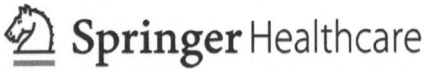

Published by Springer Healthcare Ltd, 236 Gray's Inn Road, London, WC1X 8HB, UK.

www.springerhealthcare.com

© 2014 Springer Healthcare, a part of Springer Science+Business Media.

British Library Cataloguing-in-Publication Data.

A catalogue record for this book is available from the British Library.

ISBN 978-1-907673-81-8

Although every effort has been made to ensure that drug doses and other information are presented accurately in this publication, the ultimate responsibility rests with the prescribing physician. Neither the publisher nor the authors can be held responsible for errors or for any consequences arising from the use of the information contained herein. Any product mentioned in this publication should be used in accordance with the prescribing information prepared by the manufacturers. No claims or endorsements are made for any drug or compound at present under clinical investigation.

Project editor: Tess Salazar
Designer: Joe Harvey
Production: Marina Maher
Printed in Great Britain by Latimer Trend

Contents

Author biography

Nicholas James, PhD, is Professor in Clinical Oncology and Director of the Cancer Research Unit at the University of Warwick and Honorary Consultant in Clinical Oncology at the Queen Elizabeth Hospital Birmingham. His first degree was in immunology, with first class honors. He qualified with the principal class prize in internal medicine from St Bartholomew's Hospital, London and has a PhD from Imperial College London. His postgraduate training was in London at St Bartholomew's, Hammersmith and The Royal Marsden Hospitals, with spells in Brussels and The Cancer Institute Hospital, Tokyo. He has a long-standing interest in the communication of information to patients, and founded the CancerHelp UK website in 1994 (www.cancerhelp.org.uk), now one of the largest patient websites in the world and winner of many awards. He has written numerous research papers as well as a large number of contributions to multi-author textbooks and key review articles plus *Cancer: A Very Short Introduction*, a cancer book aimed at the general public. Professor James' research interests are focused on urological cancer, from early phase to large phase 3 trials. He is chief investigator on the STAMPEDE trial, the largest prostate cancer interventional trial, which is simultaneously assessing multiple treatment options in advanced prostate cancer.

Abbreviations

ACTH	adrenocorticotropic hormone
ADT	androgen deprivation therapy
AJCC	American Joint Committee on Cancer
AR	androgen receptor
AUA	American Urological Association
BPH	benign prostatic hypertrophy
CRPC	castration-resistant prostate cancer
CZ	central zone
DHEA	dehydroepiandrosterone
DHT	dihydrotestosterone
DRE	digital rectal examination
EAU	European Association of Urology
ESMO	European Society of Medical Oncology
GnRH	gonadotropin-releasing hormone
HIFU	high-frequency focused ultrasound
HRPC	hormone-refractory prostate cancer
MDT	multidisciplinary team
MRI	magnetic resonance imaging
NICE	National Institute of Health and Care Excellence
PSA	prostate-specific antigen
PZ	peripheral zone
RP	radical prostatectomy
SRE	skeletal-related event
TNM	T, tumor; N, nodes; M, metastases
TRUS	transrectal ultrasound
TZ	transition zone

Preface

Prostate cancer is the most frequently diagnosed male cancer in the developed world and one of the leading causes of male cancer death after bowel and lung cancer. Due to both increasing rates of early diagnosis and more advanced treatment options and techniques, there are now many men who have been successfully treated for prostate cancer or who live for many years with the disease. New drugs and treatment methods will undoubtedly radically alter the way the disease is treated in the coming years. Furthermore, the rapidly decreasing costs of DNA sequencing are bringing the ability to sequence every tumor to within the realms of a routine diagnosis. The data this will yield will transform our knowledge of the biology and treatment of the disease.

This book aims to provide readers with a concise background on prostate cancer, its medical management, and new developments in the field.

Chapter 1

Epidemiology of prostate cancer

Introduction

Prostate cancer is the most commonly diagnosed cancer in men in the USA and Europe, and the second most common cause of cancer death. The incidence rates of prostate cancer vary worldwide, with the lowest rates in many parts of Asia and the highest rates in Europe, North America, and Oceania (Figure 1.1) [1,2]. Risk factors that may increase a person's chance for developing prostate cancer include older age, family history, ethnicity, high consumption of fat and red meat, and geographic location [3,4].

Incidence and prevalence

In 2008, there were an estimated 903,500 new cases of prostate cancer reported globally. There are major differences in mortality rates between countries, partially due to varying rates of clinically relevant disease or approaches to diagnosis [1]. Also, the number of deaths is more challenging to ascertain, as many men diagnosed with early prostate cancer die from causes not related to the disease.

Global variation of prostate cancer incidence and deaths may be linked to specific causes, such as diet, racial sensitivity, sun exposure, and the use of prostate-specific antigen (PSA) blood testing. Regarding sun exposure, vitamin D is involved in a range of processes, including the growth and development of cancers, bone, and glandular structures like those found in the prostate gland. Lack of exposure to sunlight for prolonged periods may thus lead to a shortage of "active" vitamin D; a study by Luscombe

N. James, *Primer on Prostate Cancer*,
DOI: 10.1007/978-1-907673-82-5_1, © Springer Healthcare 2014

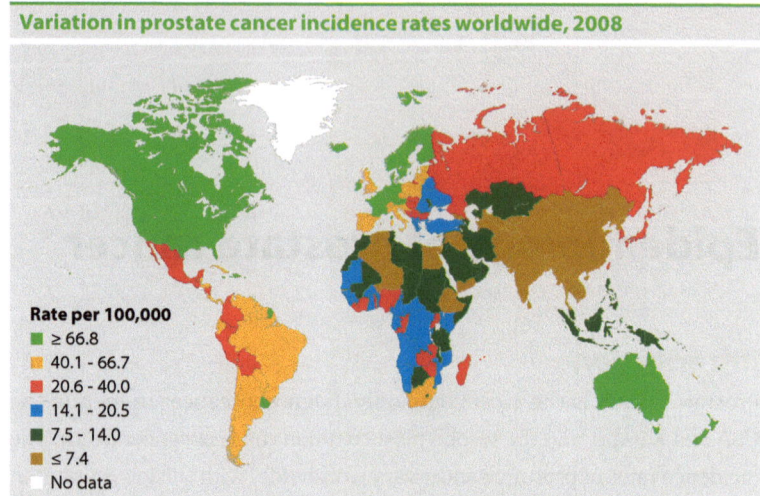

Variation in prostate cancer incidence rates worldwide, 2008

Rate per 100,000
- ≥ 66.8
- 40.1 - 66.7
- 20.6 - 40.0
- 14.1 - 20.5
- 7.5 - 14.0
- ≤ 7.4
- No data

Figure 1.1 Variation in prostate cancer incidence rates worldwide, 2008. Reproduced with permission from © American Cancer Society, 2013 [1]. All rights reserved.

and colleagues found that the risk of prostate cancer was reduced by an estimated 40% in those with the highest levels of sun exposure, as evidenced by solar skin damage and skin cancer [5]. Even in those patients who were at risk of developing prostate cancer, sun exposure appeared to delay diagnosis significantly by approximately 5 years (disease onset was at 67 years of age on average for patients with lower ultraviolet radiation exposure and at 72 years of age on average for patients with higher exposure). These effects are in part modulated by individual variations in response to the sun; however, sun exposure has a significant effect on patients with prostate cancer as well as development of the disease [5].

The use of PSA blood tests in each country also may explain variation in incidence and prevalence rates. PSA is a protein made by the prostate whose normal function is to liquefy the fluid produced during ejaculation. It is liberated in small quantities into the blood in men without cancer, but in the presence of prostate cancer as well as in other diseases affecting the prostate, larger amounts are distributed into the bloodstream, enabling the measurement of PSA to be used as both a screening and monitoring test for prostate cancer. Since the early 1990s, the test has been widely available and is used both for screening undiagnosed cancer and as a tool for monitoring the response of the cancer to treatment. Recent data from screening trials suggest that PSA testing does reduce deaths from prostate cancer [6], but in order to save one life, approximately 40 men need to have a PSA test. Also, incidence trends directly follow patterns of PSA testing, as seen in countries with higher testing rates, such as the USA, Canada, and Australia; some high-income countries, like the UK and Japan, have less dramatic incidence rates since the testing for PSA is not as common [1]. For the time being, the frequency of PSA testing worldwide is variable and largely consumer driven. Since the late 1990s, death rates have been falling at similar rates in both the USA and the UK, despite the much lower rates of PSA testing and diagnosis in the UK, suggesting that PSA testing is not the sole reason for the reduced mortality.

The prevalence of prostate cancer has also grown over the years, as more men are being successfully treated for prostate cancer or are living with the disease. The old perception that patients die "with" rather than "of" prostate cancer is at best only partially correct, with around 50% of deaths in men diagnosed with prostate cancer being attributed directly to the disease [7]. It is estimated that in the UK, there are approximately 180,000 men with prostate cancer alive up to 10 years after being diagnosed [3], and there were 217,730 prostate cancer survivors in the USA in 2010 (approximately half of the patients diagnosed survived) [1]. Worldwide numbers may be as high as 3.2 million. The issue of life after a diagnosis of prostate cancer is thus of growing importance.

References

1   American Cancer Society. *Global Cancer Facts & Figures, 2nd Edition*. Atlanta, GA: American Cancer Society, Inc.; 2011. www.cancer.org/Research/CancerFactsFigures/ GlobalCancerFactsFigures/global-cancer-facts-figures-2nd-edition.pdf. Accessed July 18, 2013.

2   Ferlay J, Shin H-R, Bray F, Forman D, Mathers C, Parkin DM. Estimates of worldwide burden of cancer in 2008: GLOBOCAN 2008. *Int J Cancer*. 2010;127:2893-2917.

3   Cancer Research UK. Prostate cancer mortality statistics. www.cancerresearchuk.org/ cancer-info/cancerstats/types/prostate/mortality/uk-prostate-cancer-mortality- statistics#age. Accessed July 18, 2013.

4   American Cancer Society. What are the risk factors for prostate cancer? www.cancer.org/ cancer/prostatecancer/detailedguide/prostate-cancer-risk-factors. Accessed July 18, 2013.

5   Luscombe CJ, Fryer AA, French ME, et al. Exposure to ultraviolet radiation: association with susceptibility and age at presentation with prostate cancer. *Lancet*. 2001;358:641-642.

6   Schröder FH, Hugosson J, Roobol MJ, et al; for the ERSPC Investigators. Screening and prostate-cancer mortality in a randomized European study. *N Engl J Med*. 2009;360:1320-1328.

7   Up to half of deaths in men with prostate cancer are directly due to the disease [press release]. London, UK: National Cancer Intelligence Network (NCIN); June 15, 2011.

Chapter 2

Clinical features and diagnosis of prostate cancer

Anatomy and function of the prostate

The prostate is a compound tubuloalveolar exocrine gland that is part of the male reproductive system (Figure 2.1) [1]. The normal adult prostate is around the size of a walnut and increases in size with age. It is situated at the base of the bladder and surrounds the urethra. The rectum sits posteriorly, allowing for the prostate to be palpated via rectal examination. The gland produces approximately 20% of the fluid produced during ejaculation; the remainder is produced by the testicles and seminal vesicles. The prostate gland contains smooth muscle fibers in addition to the glandular tissues, which contracts during ejaculation.

The glandular tissue of the prostate is dependent on androgens for normal growth and development; androgens are hormones that promotes male sex characteristics, the most common being testosterone. The secretory epithelium is pseudostratified and is supported by a fibroelastic stroma. The ductal system is connected to the prostatic urethra via the ejaculatory ducts, which are formed by the junction of the prostatic ductal systems with the vas deferens. The epithelium changes to transitional type at or near the junction of the two systems. Around the prostate is a loose fibromuscular capsule, which is sheathed in the muscles of the pelvic floor. Contraction of these muscles occurs during ejaculation [1].

N. James, *Primer on Prostate Cancer*,
DOI: 10.1007/978-1-907673-82-5_2, © Springer Healthcare 2014

Anatomy of the prostate gland

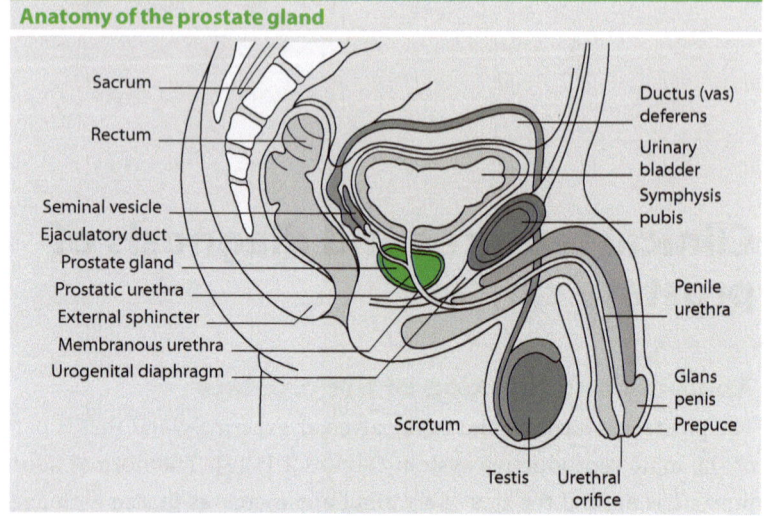

Figure 2.1 Anatomy of the prostate gland. Reproduced with permission from Theodorescu [1].

Structurally, the prostate can be divided by zone or by lobe; in clinical discussions, prostate cancer is usually described by zones. The zones described are:

- Peripheral zone (PZ): comprises of the posterior part of the gland surrounding the distal urethra. Between 80–85% of cancers arise in the PZ [2].
- Central zone (CZ): surrounds the ejaculatory ducts. Only approximately 5–10% of cancers arise in the CZ [2].
- Transition zone (TZ): surrounds the proximal urethra. The TZ enlarges throughout life and is the part of the gland where benign prostatic hypertrophy (BPH) occurs in later life. Approximately 10–15% of cancers originate from the TZ [2].
- Anterior fibromuscular zone or stroma: forms the entire anterior surface of the prostate as a thick, nonglandular apron, shielding from view the anterior surface of the three glandular regions [3].

The zonal system more closely describes the functional and pathological processes within the prostate gland. The zonal system is illustrated in Figure 2.2 [3].

Zonal anatomy of the prostate gland

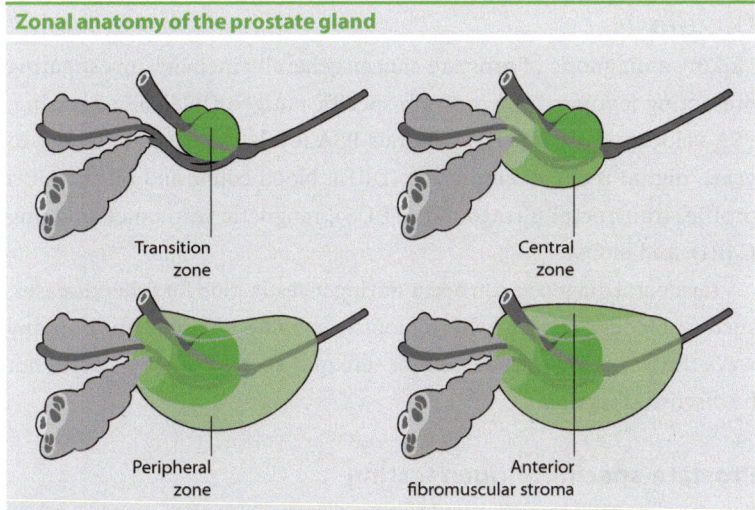

Figure 2.2 Zonal anatomy of the prostate gland. Reproduced with permission from Taylor and Albertsen [3].

Symptoms of prostate cancer

Prostate cancer symptoms can include erectile dysfunction, blood in the semen, pain in the lower back, hips, and/or upper thighs, urinary problems, or enlargement of the prostate. Enlargement of the prostate can lead to obstruction with reduced flow, hesitancy, post-micturition dribbling, or even retention, bleeding, and/or infection. An overlapping problem set appears from urinary irritation. It is important to point out that all of these symptoms occur in men with BPH as well as other disorders arising from other parts of the urinary system. Clinicians should perform standard examinations and testing to make the most appropriate diagnosis while ruling out other possible diseases.

Symptoms from metastasis

Most commonly, symptoms from metastasis occur from bone secondaries, causing pain or fracture. Occasionally, patients will present with nodal enlargement causing palpable masses, lymphedema, or venous thromboembolism.

Diagnosis

Making a diagnosis of prostate cancer generally includes investigating presenting features from prostate-specific antigen (PSA) blood testing, PSA velocity (how much a patient's PSA levels increase from year to year), digital rectal examination (DRE), blood count and biochemical profile, transrectal ultrasound (TRUS), magnetic resonance imaging (MRI), and biopsy.

Incidental diagnosis can occur during investigation for other diseases, such as bladder cancer, where biopsies may be undertaken. In many ways the issues are the same as for screen-detected cancer and will not be discussed further.

Prostate-specific antigen testing

Prostate cancer screening is done in part through the use of the PSA blood tests and is often combined with a DRE. As previously discussed in Chapter 1, the rate of PSA screenings vary from country to country, and studies have shown conflicting results as to whether PSA screening is useful when determining if biopsies are needed for patients with suspected disease [4,5]. PSA levels should be evaluated in line with other diagnostic techniques when managing a patient with prostate cancer [6,7]. Not all low or high PSA levels will necessarily indicate that a patient has or does not have prostate cancer, as PSA levels are organ specific and not cancer specific. Clinicians should administer and evaluate PSA levels with caution to avoid unnecessary subsequent biopsies and possible adverse events. Despite the inherent risk of PSA testing, PSA levels still may indicate a patient's risk for prostate cancer (Table 2.1), although

Low prostate-specific antigen levels and the risk of prostate cancer	
Prostate-specific antigen level (ng/mL)	Risk of prostate cancer
0–0.5	6.6%
0.6–1	10.1%
1.1–2	17.0%
2.1–3	23.9%
3.1–4	26.9%

Table 2.1 Low prostate-specific antigen levels and the risk of prostate cancer. Reproduced with permission from © Elsevier, Heidenreich et al, 2013 [7]. All rights reserved.

those chances are small and should be evaluated with other diagnostic measures in mind [6,7].

Digital rectal examination

DREs are performed by a clinician physically examining the prostate via the rectum for any bumps, enlargements, or suspicious hard areas. As most prostate cancers are located in the PZ, a DRE may detect cancers in this zone when its volume is approximately 0.2 mL or larger; about 18% of patients with prostate cancer can be diagnosed by a DRE regardless of PSA levels [7]. As reported in the European Association of Urology (EAU) guidelines, when PSA levels of up to 2 ng/mL are taken into account, a suspect DRE has a positive predictive value of 5–30%; additionally, a DRE can indicate whether a prostate biopsy is recommended for a patient, especially in more aggressive cases [7].

However, like PSA blood testing, DREs are not absolutely conclusive. The American Urological Association (AUA) 2013 guidelines could not find evidence to support the continued use of DREs for first-line screening due to their lack of sensitivity and the high possibility of missing early prostate cancer tumors, which may not be felt during the examination [6]. Nevertheless, the AUA panel acknowledged the standard practice of DREs, and given that prostate cancer could be found with DREs, still suggests that the examination used in conjunction with other diagnostic tests could be helpful when screening patients for prostate cancer [6].

Transrectal ultrasound

A TRUS is performed by inserting a small probe in the patient's rectum; this probe emits sound waves into the patient's prostate that echoes back to the probe to ultimately create video images of the prostate. The TRUS can sometimes detect tumors that may not have been detected by a DRE, and it may also give clinicians a better idea of PSA density, which can help distinguish between BPH and prostate cancer. It should be noted that TRUS may not always be able to distinguish between normal tissue and cancer tissue; however, TRUS is an important imaging test when prostate needle biopsies are to be performed, as it gives a visual location of where possible tumors might be located.

Magnetic resonance imaging

For patients who are likely to have low-risk disease (no symptoms, low PSA [<10 ng/mL], low PSA velocity), there is a growing body of opinion that multiparametric MRI should be performed ahead of biopsy, with the possibility that patients with a low risk of cancer on imaging may be offered observation with no initial biopsy [8]. The rationale is that biopsy artifacts on an MRI persist for 3–6 months, making accurate staging difficult post-biopsy. Using multiple MRI sequences on a "clean" prostate allows for an increasingly accurate estimate of the risk of clinically significant disease. Given the low risk of death from early prostate cancer, the reduction in morbidity from avoiding biopsy is attractive as it also prevents the trauma of a cancer diagnosis.

Biopsy

A comprehensive review of the patient's history, age, ethnicity, heredity, comorbidities, and their results from PSA blood tests, DREs, and imaging tests should all be evaluated before determining if a biopsy is needed [4,7]. High PSA levels in particular should not be the sole reason to perform biopsies given the inconclusive correlation between high PSA levels and actual presentation of prostate cancer [5]. PSA levels should be validated by repeat PSA tests [7] and supported by suspicious DREs, imaging results, and the patient's overall history and risk factors [4–7].

Prostate cancer biopsies can be performed by transrectal, perineal, or transurethral method. As mentioned above, biopsies can be guided by TRUS to give clinicians a visual location of possible tumors. Once the suspicious tissue is extracted, the patient's possible prostate cancer can be examined pathologically. While biopsies and an analysis of the tumor histology can allow clinicians to appropriately determine the patient's disease and its severity, the biopsy procedure can also lead to adverse events, such as infection, bleeding, and urinary difficulties, and clinicians should take extra caution to avoid such complications [5]. In addition, with the growing use of MRI prebiopsy, targeted biopsy (usually transperineal using MRI derived information) is increasingly used.

Pathology and the Gleason system

The Gleason system was developed by Dr Donald Gleason in the early 1970s and has become the preferred histological grading system of prostate cancer [2]. The Gleason system is based upon the degree of loss of the normal glandular tissue architecture (Figure 2.3) [9]. Biopsies are graded from 1–5 and then an aggregate score incorporating the principal and major secondary score is produced (eg, 3 + 4 = 7). Scores conventionally tend to be grouped into the following broader risk categories:

- 1–5: low-grade prostate cancer
- 6–7: intermediate-grade cancer (most prostate cancers fall into this group)
- 8–10: high-grade cancer

Increasingly, however, pathologists are reluctant to use Gleason grades of 1 or 2, making 3 effectively the lowest grade cancer score. A Gleason score of 3 + 3 is thus now regarded as low risk, 3 + 4 and 4 + 3 as intermediate risk, and 8–10 as high risk. Care must therefore be taken when comparing recent with older data due to this grade migration.

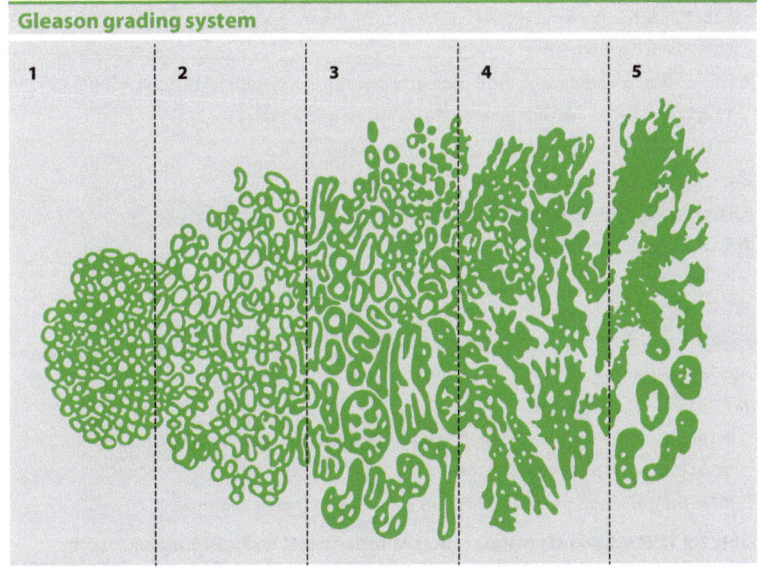

Gleason grading system

| 1 | 2 | 3 | 4 | 5 |

Figure 2.3 Gleason grading system. This illustration exemplifies the Gleason grading system, with five basic tissue patterns associated with five tumor grades. Reproduced with permission from Huang et al [9].

Staging

Generally, conventional staging is done using the American Joint Committee on Cancer (AJCC) TNM classification system (Tables 2.2 and 2.3) [2], which is based on:

- the evaluation of the primary tumor (T category),
- whether the cancer has spread to regional (nearby) lymph nodes (N category),
- whether there is evidence of distant metastasis (M category),

TNM staging of prostate cancer
Clinical evaluation of the primary tumor (T)
TX: Cannot evaluate the primary tumor
T0: No evidence of tumor
T1: Tumor present, but not detectable clinically or with imaging
T1a: Tumor was incidentally found in <5% of prostate tissue resected (for other reasons)
T1b: Tumor was incidentally found in >5% of prostate tissue resected
T1c: Tumor was found in a needle biopsy performed due to an elevated serum PSA
T2: Tumor can be felt (palpated) on examination, but has not spread outside the prostate
T2a: Tumor is in half or less than half of one of two lobes of the prostate gland
T2b: Tumor is in more than half of one lobe, but not both
T2c: Tumor is in both lobes
T3: Tumor has spread through the prostatic capsule (if it is only partway through, it is still **T2**)
T3a: Tumor has spread through the capsule on one or both sides
T3b: Tumor has invaded one or both seminal vesicles
T4: Tumor has invaded other nearby structures
Clinical evaluation of the regional lymph nodes (N)
NX: Cannot evaluate the regional lymph nodes
N0: There has been no spread to the regional lymph nodes
N1: There has been spread to the regional lymph nodes
Evaluation of distant metastasis (M)
M0: There is no distant metastasis
M1: There is distant metastasis
M1a: The cancer has spread to lymph nodes beyond the regional ones
M1b: The cancer has spread to bone
M1c: The cancer has spread to other sites (regardless of bone involvement)

Table 2.2 TNM staging of prostate cancer. M, metastasis; N, nodes; PSA, prostate-specific antigen; T, tumor. Reproduced with permission from © American Joint Committee on Cancer, 2013 [2]. All rights reserved. Additional information provided by Heidenreich et al [7].

- the PSA levels at the time of diagnosis, and
- the Gleason score based on a biopsy.

The use of additional staging/diagnostic tests should match the severity of disease as determined by the biopsy and prostate imaging (TRUS or MRI). Based on clinical experience, patients with low-risk disease (PSA <10 ng/mL, Gleason 3 + 3 or 3 + 4 if aged >70–75 years) probably need no further imaging. The likelihood of metastasis increases in patients with intermediate- and high-risk disease, and in these cases full staging is justified, with cross-sectional abdominal and pelvic imaging at a minimum as well as an isotope bone scan. In practice, it is in the author's opinion that it is helpful to define prostate cancer by risk group when evaluating the patient (see Table 2.4 for other classification methods) [7,10–13]; multiple risk groups may overlap, but the analysis will provide a more comprehensive view of the patient's cancer.

American Joint Committee on Cancer anatomic stage/prognostic groups					
Group	T	N	M	PSA	Gleason
I	T1a–c	N0	M0	PSA<10	Gleason ≤6
	T2a	N0	M0	PSA<10	Gleason ≤6
	T1–2a	N0	M0	PSA X	Gleason X
IIA	T1a–c	N0	M0	PSA<20	Gleason 7
	T1a–c	N0	M0	PSA≥10<20	Gleason ≤6
	T2a	N0	M0	PSA≥10<20	Gleason ≤6
	T2a	N0	M0	PSA<20	Gleason 7
	T2b	N0	M0	PSA<20	Gleason ≤7
	T2b	N0	M0	PSA X	Gleason X
IIB	T2c	N0	M0	Any PSA	Any Gleason
	T1–2	N0	M0	PSA ≥20	Any Gleason
	T1–2	N0	M0	Any PSA	Gleason ≥8
III	T3a–b	N0	M0	Any PSA	Any Gleason
IV	T4	N0	M0	Any PSA	Any Gleason
	Any T	N1	M0	Any PSA	Any Gleason
	Any T	Any N	M1	Any PSA	Any Gleason

Table 2.3 American Joint Committee on Cancer anatomic stage/prognostic groups. When either PSA or Gleason is not available, grouping should be determined by T stage and/or either PSA or Gleason as available. M, metastasis; N, nodes; PSA, prostate-specific antigen; T, tumor. Reproduced with permission from © AJCC Cancer Staging Manual, 2013 [2]. All rights reserved.

Categorization by risk group

Classification	Definition
European Association of Urology [7]	
High-risk, localized prostate cancer	cT3a *or* Gleason score 8–10 *or* PSA >20 ng/mL
	T2c *or* Gleason score >7 *or* PSA >20 ng/mL
Locally advanced prostate cancer	cT3a
	T3–4, N0, M0
	T3–4, any N *or* any T, N1
European Society of Medical Oncology [10]	
High-risk localized (also locally advanced disease)	T3–4 *or* Gleason score >7 *or* PSA >20 ng/mL
National Comprehensive Cancer Center [11]	
High-risk localized	T3a *or* Gleason score 8–10 *or* PSA >20 ng/mL
Locally advanced/very high	T3b–T4
National Collaborating Centre for Cancer/National Institute of Health and Care Excellence [12]	
High-risk localized	T3–T4 *or* Gleason score 8–10 *or* PSA >20 ng/mL
Locally advanced prostate cancer	T3–T4, any N, M
STAMPEDE trial [13]	
High risk, nonmetastatic	Any 2 from: T3–4, Gleason score 8-10, PSA >40 ng/mL

Table 2.4 Categorization by risk group. M, metastasis; N, nodes; PSA, prostate-specific antigen; T, tumor. Adapted from Heidenrech et al [7], Horwich et al [10], National Comprehensive Cancer Center [11], National Collaborating Centre for Cancer [12], and STAMPEDE Trial [13].

References

1   Theodorescu D. Prostate cancer, clinical oncology. In: Schwab M, ed. *Encyclopedic Reference of Cancer*. Berlin, Germany: Springer-Verlag; 2001:720-727.

2   American Joint Committee on Cancer. *AJCC Cancer Staging Manual*. 7th ed. New York, NY: Springer Science+Business Media; 2010.

3   Taylor JA, Albertsen PC. Benign and malignant disease of the prostate. In: Rosenthal RA, Zenilman ME, Katlic MR, eds. *Principles and Practice of Geriatric Surgery*. 2nd ed. New York, NY: Springer Science+Business Media; 2011:1069-1082.

4   Descotes J-L, Legeais D, Gauchez A-S, Long J-A, Rambeaud J-J. PSA measurement following prostatectomy: an unexpected error. *Anticancer Res*. 2007;27:1149-1150.

5   Basch E, Oliver TK, Vickers A, et al. Screening for prostate cancer with prostate-specific antigen testing: American Society of Clinical Oncology provisional clinical opinion. *J Clin Oncol*. 2012;30:3020-3025.

6   Carter HB, Albertsen PC, Barry MJ, et al. Early detection of prostate cancer: AUA guideline. www.auanet.org/common/pdf/education/clinical-guidance/Prostate-Cancer-Detection.pdf. Accessed July 18, 2013.

7   Heidenreich A, Bellmunt J, Bolla M, et al. EAU guidelines on prostate cancer. Part I: screening, diagnosis, and treatment of clinically localised disease. *Eur Urol*. 2011;59:61-71.

8   Gupta RT, Kauffman CR, Polascik TJ, Taneja SS, Rosenkrantz AB. The state of prostate MRI in 2013. *Oncology (Williston Park)*. 2013;27:262-270.

9   Huang PW, Lee C-H, Lin P-L. Classifying pathological prostate images by fractal analysis. In: Chatterjee A, Siarry P, eds. *Computational Intelligence in Image Processing*. Heidelberg, Germany: Springer-Verlag Berlin Heidelberg; 2013:253-263.

10 Horwich A, Parker C, Bangma C, Kataja V; on behalf of the ESMO Guidelines Working Group. Prostate cancer: ESMO Clinical Practice Guidelines for diagnosis, treatment and follow-up. *Ann Oncol*. 2010;21(suppl 5):v129-v133.

11 National Comprehensive Cancer Center (NCCN). NCCN clinical practice guidelines in oncology (NCCN Guideline®): prostate cancer. www.nccn.org/professionals/physician_gls/pdf/prostate. pdf. Accessed July 18, 2013.

12 National Collaborating Centre for Cancer. Prostate cancer: diagnosis and treatment. 2008. www.nice.org.uk/nicemedia/live/11924/39687/39687.pdf. Accessed July 18, 2013.

13 STAMPEDE: Systemic Therapy in Advancing or Metastatic Prostate Cancer: Evaluation of Drug Efficacy: a multi-stage multi-arm randomised controlled trial. www.clinicaltrials.gov/ct2/show/study/NCT00268476. Accessed July 18, 2013.

Chapter 3

Management of patients with prostate cancer

Overview of current developments in the field

Various new drugs and treatment techniques have become available in recent years for patients with prostate cancer. In addition, there is a growing realization that many patients with low-risk disease can be safely monitored initially with deferred treatment, if needed. These developments in therapies also coincide with advancements made in imaging technology, which may allow for better identification of those patients with potential life-threatening disease and other patients strictly in need of monitoring for indolent disease.

Currently, men diagnosed with prostate cancer often pass through a long disease process that starts with localized or locally advanced disease, prostate-specific antigen (PSA) relapse, hormone therapy followed by development of what is now termed castration-resistant prostate cancer (CRPC), previously termed hormone-refractory prostate cancer (HRPC). Until recently, there were few treatments for CRPC. Over the last 10 years, there has been a procession of new drugs showing a survival advantage in patients with CRPC. Furthermore, many of these agents are from different drug classes and may be expected to confer at least a partially additive benefit when administered in combination.

Additionally, the rapidly decreasing costs of DNA sequencing are bringing the ability to sequence every tumor to within the realms of routine diagnosis. These data will transform our knowledge of the

N. James, *Primer on Prostate Cancer*,
DOI: 10.1007/978-1-907673-82-5_3, © Springer Healthcare 2014

biology of the disease and allow more rational treatment choices based on tumor biology.

Whether the aim of treatment is to cure, prolong life, or provide for palliation of symptoms, a range of approaches are available and may be used either alone or in combination, depending on disease status. These treatment approaches can include surgery, radiotherapy, hormone therapy, and/or chemotherapy. Decisions should be reviewed on a regular basis by the multidisciplinary team (MDT) and treatment should be adapted in response to side effects and tumor response. Current European and American treatment guidelines can be found in Table 3.1 (see page 20) [1–6]. The following sections in this chapter will describe the available major therapeutic options, including those listed above, deferring treatment, biologics, and treatment for metastatic disease. Guidelines and clinical opinions will vary on specific treatment methods, as there is not a consensus on one optimal treatment plan at the time of this book's publication. Also, note that although many of these guidelines were published recently, the rapid changes in treatment options make all of them at least partly out-of-date.

Multidisciplinary team

Since treatment of prostate cancer is complex, especially with new technologies available, decisions are now increasingly being made by MDTs in major healthcare systems rather than by individual doctors. Specifically in the UK, decision-making made by an MDT is now mandatory if the hospital is to receive reimbursement for cancer therapy. Typically, these teams are comprised of surgeons, radiation and medical oncologists, radiologists, pathologists, and specialist nurses. The MDT should aim to review the staging information prior to consultation with the patient in order to form a consensus on the most appropriate treatment options for a patient (see Chapter 2).

Deferring treatment

Deferring treatment for some patients may be the suitable option if they are in a low-risk group or are at intermediate-risk but are not suitable for or do not want radical treatment [1,3,4]. By deferring treatment, men in these risk groups can avoid unnecessary treatment-related complications, especially since their disease may not progress [1,4]. Also, by clinicians deferring treatment through "watchful waiting" or "active surveillance," they may be able to observe the patient's disease for a longer time period, and thus allow for more specific treatment plans for the patient [4]. Watchful waiting refers to when the MDT and patient agree to postpone definitive treatment and to focus on palliative care, including transurethral resection or urinary tract obstruction [1,4]. Active surveillance tends to focus on closely monitoring patients rather than watchful waiting. If the patient's disease is likely to progress, the MDT should provide precise treatment plans, which the patient should be educated on and accept before pursuing; however, if the patient's disease is not likely to progress, the MDT and patient should focus on reducing possible treatment-related complications [4].

Role of surgery

The first question to be addressed in patients with localized disease is whether surgery is indicated and feasible. Decisions need to take account the patient's overall fitness, life expectancy, and preferences regarding treatment, and there should be discussion of the risks and benefits of surgery as compared to other treatment options.

Benefits of surgery may include:

- curing the disease; and
- obtaining clarity regarding outcomes (eg, clear surgical margins, low postoperative PSA levels, and lower risk of relapse due to detailed pathological staging information).

Potential downsides to surgery may include:

- risks of incontinence and impotence;
- incomplete resection with need for further local radiotherapy;
- wound healing (eg, physical healing, time off from work); and/or
- metastatic relapse.

Surgical options for prostate cancer treatment are discussed below. Prostatectomy is the most common surgery, and can be done manually, laparoscopically, or with robotic assistance.

Summary of prostate cancer treatment guidelines (continues opposite)

	Clinically localized disease	Advanced disease
European Association of Urology (EAU) [1,2]	*RP* • Patients with low- and intermediate-risk localized prostate cancer (cT1a–T2b, Gleason score 2–7, and PSA ≤20) and a life expectancy >10 years *Definitive radiation therapy* • Patients with locally advanced prostate cancer T3–T4 N0 M0 and/or high-risk disease, combined with hormonal therapy for up to 3 years • Immediate postoperative use after RP for patients with pathologic tumor stage T3 N0 M0	*Hormonal therapy* • GnRH agonists • Anti-androgens • Short-term use: reduction of risk of the "flare-up" phenomenon in patients with advanced metastatic disease who are to receive a GnRH agonist • Primary monotherapy as an alternative to castration
European Society for Medical Oncology (ESMO) [3]	Options based on either surgery or on radiotherapy should be considered and each therapy's possible adverse effects discussed with the patient *Radiation therapy* • If used as the sole treatment modality, dose escalation to ≥74 Gy can be used • For salvage radiotherapy following RP that treats only biochemical evidence of prostate cancer, a dose ≥66 Gy is recommended *Radiation therapy + hormone therapy* • In localized intermediate-risk disease, moderate-dose radiotherapy (<70 Gy) should be combined with 6 months of ADT	• Patients with locally advanced prostate cancer to be treated with hormonal therapy alone can be given intermittent androgen deprivation • Hormone therapy can also be used with radiotherapy for ≥6 months (≥24 months for high-risk patients) • RP for locally advanced T3–T4 disease should be done only after careful staging and discussion
American Urological Association (AUA) [4–6]	*Active surveillance, interstitial prostate brachytherapy, external beam radiotherapy, RP* • Low-risk and intermediate-risk patients (any of these options) The above measures are also treatment options for high-risk patients, but recurrence rates are high. RP may lower chance of recurrence, and radiotherapy may be more effective if used in combination with hormonal therapy	

Table 3.1 Summary of European and American prostate cancer treatment guidelines (continues opposite). ADT, androgen deprivation therapy; GnRH, gonadotropin-releasing hormone; M, metastasis; N, node; PSA, prostate-specific antigen; RP, radical prostatectomy; T, tumor. Adapted from Heidenreich et al [1], Mottet et al [2], Horwich et al [3], American Urological Association [4], Thompson et al [5], Cookson et al [6].

Summary of prostate cancer treatment guidelines (continued)

Relapsing disease	Castration-resistant prostate cancer
• GnRH agonists/ orchiectomy or bicalutamide 150 mg/day when hormonal therapy is indicated • Systemic relapse: early ADT • Local recurrences: salvage radiation therapy with 64–66 Gy at a PSA serum level ≤0.5 ng/mL	• Docetaxel 75 mg/m^2 q3wk, with cabazitaxel as second-line therapy • In patients with symptomatic osseous metastases, docetaxel or mitoxantrone with prednisone or hydrocortisone
• Immediate ADT for pN1 patients after RP who have a high risk for progression • Radical locoregional therapy for N1 M0 patients who are suitable for aggressive management treatment	*Nonmetastatic* • Lifelong ADT • Patients who progress on ADT: androgen-receptor inhibitors, estrogen, ketoconazole (now withdrawn in many countries), steroids, or withdrawal of ADT *Metastatic* • Docetaxel, with cabazitaxel, abiraterone, enzalutamide, and radium Ra 223 dichloride as second-line agents • Additional hormone manipulations if short-term responses are needed
• Restaging with PSA recurrence can be considered • Salvage therapy: disease has recurred after RP but there is no evidence of distant metastatic disease	*Nonmetastatic* • Observation with continued ADT • If patient is unwilling to accept observation, consider steroid + ketoconazole, flutamide, bicalutamide, or nilutamide • Do not treat with systemic chemotherapy or immunotherapy *Metastatic* • Asymptomatic or minimally symptomatic, with good performance status and docetaxel-naïve: docetaxel, abiraterone + prednisone, or sipuleucel-T • Symptomatic, with good performance status and docetaxel-naïve: docetaxel • Symptomatic, with poor performance status and docetaxel-naïve: abiraterone + prednisone, steroid + ketoconazole, or radionuclide therapy • Symptomatic, with good performance status and prior docetaxel treatment: abiraterone + prednisone, cabazitaxel, enzalutamide, steroid + ketoconazole, or retreatment with docetaxel • Symptomatic, with poor performance status and prior docetaxel treatment: palliative care, abiraterone + prednisone, enzalutamide, steroid + ketoconazole, or radionuclide therapy

Figure 3.1 shows the relative roles of surgery, radiotherapy, and monitoring in nonmetastatic, node negative disease.

Open radical prostatectomy

Open radical prostatectomy, the complete removal of the prostate through direct manual means by the surgeon, was pioneered by Patrick Walsh at The Johns Hopkins School of Medicine [7]. Despite the development of minimally invasive techniques, there is still a need for open radical prostatectomy as it has potential advantages in certain circumstances, such as nerve sparing. With modern enhanced recovery techniques, the typical length of stay is around two days and blood loss is minimal. The direct access to the prostate is potentially an advantage in nerve-sparing operations and the author's own center (Queen Elizabeth Hospital Birmingham) has reverted back to open radical prostatectomy for this indication.

Laparoscopic radical prostatectomy

Laparoscopic radical prostatectomy is a minimally invasive surgery, involving few incisions, to remove the whole prostate. It is technically

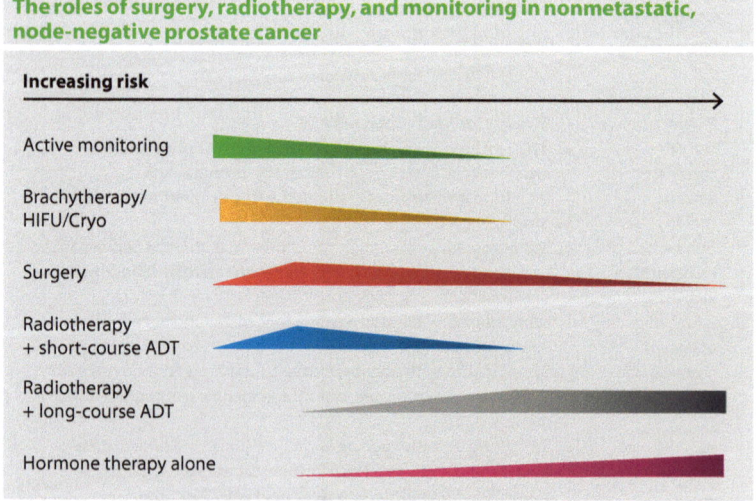

Figure 3.1 The roles of surgery, radiotherapy, and monitoring in nonmetastatic, node-negative prostate cancer. ADT, androgen deprivation therapy; Cryo, cryotherapy; HIFU, high-frequency focused ultrasound.

challenging to master due to the lever effect of the instruments and hence both operation times and the total learning curve are longer than with open radical prostatectomy. This is compensated by shorter inpatient postoperative stays and faster recovery to full activity due to the absence of the abdominal wound that results from open prostatectomy procedures.

Robot-assisted prostatectomy

In the USA and many parts of the world, laparoscopic radical prostatectomy is often being performed by robot-assisted surgery using the *da Vinci*® Surgical System (Intuitive Surgical, Inc., Sunnyvale, CA, USA), commonly known as the da Vinci robot. This maintains the advantages of laparoscopic radical prostatectomy and has a much more rapid learning curve, plus it provides for a 3D, magnified field of vision. No randomized trial data exist and the currently available data do not support the superiority of one modality over another [8]. The main drawbacks of the da Vinci robot are its substantial cost and the increased maintenance that is required compared with open or other laparoscopic surgical systems. At present, this is compounded by there being only a single manufacturer.

Pelvic lymphadenectomy

Extended pelvic lymphadenectomy is often done at the same time as a radical prostatectomy. It involves regional dissection and draining of the lymph nodes beyond what is typically done during standard pelvic lymphadenectomy (the external iliac artery and obturator fossa), to include the internal iliac, common iliac, and presacral lymph nodes [9]. One study found it to be beneficial in patients with a preoperative serum PSA >10.5 ng/mL and a biopsy Gleason and Ritchie sum >6 [9]. It is recommended in both the EU and USA for patients with intermediate- or high-risk prostate cancer [1,4].

Surgically based treatments

In addition to conventional surgery, there are evolving techniques that are usually administered by surgeons, in particular high-frequency focused ultrasound (HIFU) and cryotherapy, discussed below.

High-frequency focused ultrasound

HIFU is a minimally invasive technique that uses high-energy sound waves, which are focused via a transrectal probe to locally ablate cancer in the prostate. The treatment dates back to the 1940s but only became used for prostate cancer in the mid-1990s. The technique is only suitable for organ-confined disease and low-risk patients or for patients with local failure following radiotherapy. There are no randomized trials comparing HIFU to surgery, radiotherapy, or active monitoring.

Cryotherapy

As with HIFU, cryotherapy is a locally image-guided procedure that ablates cancerous tissue without the use of ionizing radiation. The treatment works by the insertion of needles into the prostate, which are then cooled with liquid nitrogen, followed by a time interval to allow for thawing; the freeze-thaw damage to cells can be monitored via a transrectal ultrasound probe (see Figure 3.2). A urinary catheter containing warmed saline is used to protect the urethra from thermal injury. Neither HIFU nor cryotherapy treatment is routinely available in the UK due to concerns about possible side effects and the lack of comparative efficacy studies; similarly, the AUA stated that due to limited data available, a recommendation for HIFU and cryotherapy cannot be made yet [4]. Side

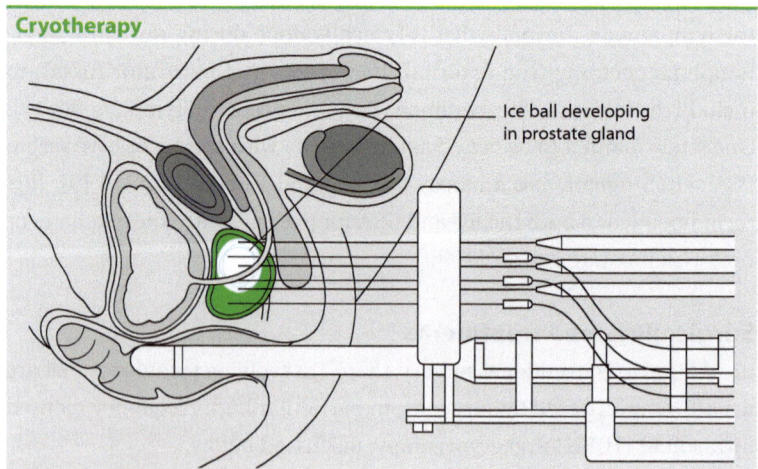

Cryotherapy

Ice ball developing
in prostate gland

Figure 3.2 Cryotherapy.

effects include erectile dysfunction, pain and swelling of the scrotum and penis, hematuria, urinary incontinence, frequent urination, and difficulty or painful urination [10].

Radiotherapy

Radiotherapy is one of the mainstays of prostate cancer treatment. Forms of radiotherapy include external beam radiotherapy and brachytherapy. As summarized earlier in this chapter, the role of radiotherapy in localized disease has to be considered in relation to other modalities, such as surgery or monitoring, and to the disease stage.

Nodal disease

Prostate cancer can spread to regional lymph nodes with increasing frequency as adverse disease characteristics increase; however, current imaging technology still often fails to identify pathologically involved nodes. Trials of nodal radiotherapy have, therefore, been conducted in high-risk, radiologically node-negative patients. The most recent of these, the French GETUG-01 trial, failed to show any benefit from nodal radiotherapy in the highest-risk cohort [11]. To date, no randomized trials have been carried out in radiologically node-positive patients.

External beam radiotherapy

Most radiotherapy is delivered as external beam therapy via a linear accelerator (linac). High-energy (megavoltage) beams are focused into the patient from multiple directions to deliver the dose to the target volume; areas given external bean radiotherapy include the prostate and the base of the seminal vesicles, plus a margin around these structures to allow for microscopic local spread and organ movement during treatment. Modern linacs are equipped with multileaf collimation systems, which allow beams to be custom shaped to the target volume in a dynamic fashion that can change during treatment; this is also known as intensity-modulated radiation therapy. In addition, on-board imaging systems on linacs allow the target to be verified if necessary on a daily basis and adjustments made to ensure conformity of delivered treatment to the pretherapy plan. This radiotherapy can reduce treatment-related toxicity, but may increase the risk of relapse or second malignancy due to larger volumes of normal tissues being irradiated to lower doses.

Brachytherapy

In brachytherapy, small radioactive seeds are implanted into the prostate under transrectal ultrasound image guidance, delivering a high dose of radiation directly to the prostate with little spread to surrounding tissues (Figure 3.3) [12]. This latter feature is also a potential drawback, as periprostatic spread will not be treated, unlike with external beam radiotherapy where a periprostatic margin can be included. Brachytherapy is thus only suitable for lower-risk, prostate-confined disease, for which there are several other treatment options. A variant form of brachytherapy uses implanted catheters that can be connected to a high-dose rate brachytherapy device, which loads sources into the catheters for short duration treatments of 15–20 minutes, typically twice in a day repeated weekly for a total of six treatments. This has the advantage of no permanent implant, a much shorter duration of therapy than standard external beam radiation therapy, and shorter operative recovery time than surgery. High-dose rate brachytherapy is used in some centers in

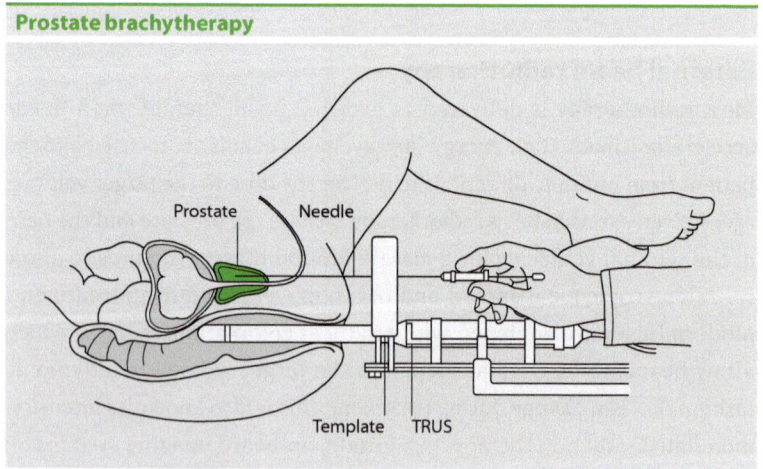

Prostate brachytherapy

Figure 3.3 Prostate brachytherapy. TRUS, transrectal ultrasound. Reproduced with permission from Theodorescu [12].

combination with external beam treatments for higher-risk cases. There are no large randomized trials comparing any of the brachytherapy techniques against standard external beam therapy or surgery.

CyberKnife® Robotic Radiosurgery System

The CyberKnife® Robotic Radiosurgery System (Accuray Incorporated, Sunnyvale, CA, USA) is a conventional linac mounted on a robot arm, which allows for multiple, narrow, noncoplanar beams to target small volumes very precisely. The technology uses implanted fiducial markers and real-time imaging to track the location of the tumor during the treatment. Typically, small numbers of large fractions (termed hypofractionation) are used rather than the multiweek courses used for conventional radiotherapy. Patients experience minimal side effects during this outpatient procedure, and the recovery time is generally quick. Side effects may include constipation, urinary retention, incontinence, erectile dysfunction, blood in the stool, and injury to rectal wall, bladder wall, or nearby tissue [13]. Again, there are no randomized comparisons against other major treatment modalities so at present the precise role of this technique is undefined. As for brachytherapy, there is the potential concern that the higher accuracy may lead to the use of smaller periprostatic margins (to keep toxicity down) and in turn a risk of edge recurrences. The precise dose equivalents of the hypofractionated schedules used on CyberKnife when compared to longer conventional fractionations are at this time also unclear.

Hormone therapy

Androgens are male sex hormones and include several steroids, such as testosterone, which is the main circulating androgen in the human body. Most prostate cancer cells rely on testosterone for their growth and therapeutic approaches that reduce testosterone levels or block its action in prostate cancer cells (termed hormone therapy or androgen deprivation therapy [ADT]) are a standard treatment method for advanced prostate cancer. Examples of hormone therapy in prostate cancer are summarized in Table 3.2. Androgen pathways and therapeutic targets therein are summarized in Figure 3.4.

Targets of hormone therapy

Targets	Examples of prostate cancer therapy
Block synthesis of regulator of hormone	GnRH agonists and antagonists such as goserelin, leuprolide, triptorelin
Block binding of secreted hormone to androgen receptor	Bicalutamide, enzalutamide, cyproterone acetate
Block post-receptor effects	Enzalutamide
Block synthesis of hormone	CYP17 inhibitors (abiraterone)
Add alternative hormones to alter environment	Diethylstilboestrol, dexamethasone

Table 3.2 Targets of hormone therapy. GnRH, gonadotropin-releasing hormone.

Androgen pathways and therapeutic targets

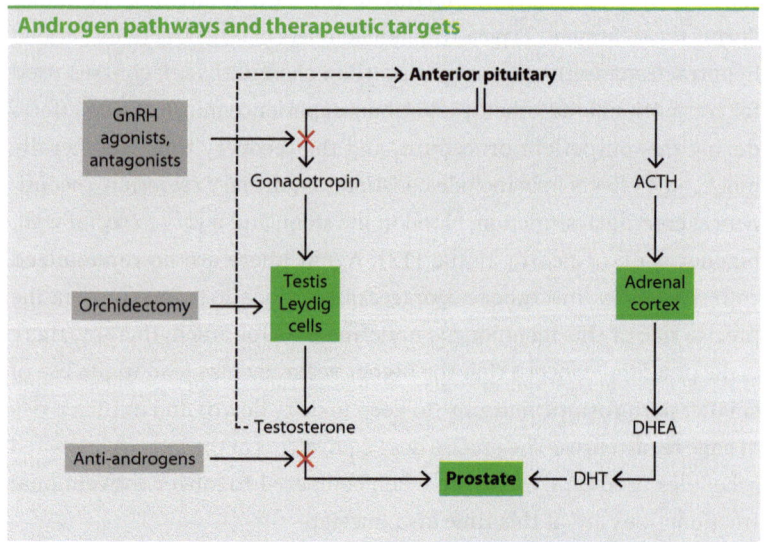

Figure 3.4 Androgen pathways and therapeutic targets. ACTH, adrenocorticotropic hormone; DHEA, dehydroepiandrosterone; DHT, dihydrotestosterone; GnRH, gonadotropin-releasing hormone.

Hormone therapy has been a mainstay of prostate cancer treatment since the seminal studies of Huggins and Hodges published in 1941 that demonstrated substantial and prolonged remissions from prostate cancer with the use of either surgical castration or estrogen therapy [14]. Patterns of hormone therapy use vary with disease stage and also between countries.

Diethylstilbestrol was the first example of a successful drug treatment for advanced cancer, and while it is now supplanted in this role by newer agents, it remains in use 70 years later. Although responses to hormone therapy may be dramatic and last for many years, they are rarely curative and typically last for only 18–24 months, depending on disease stage. This period after failure of initial hormone therapy has been known by many terms over the years, including androgen-independent prostate cancer, HRPC, and most recently CRPC. Before the approval of abiraterone in 2011, agents primarily blocked testosterone synthesis or its action on prostate tissues, including cancer. These treatments may thus be grouped together as "castration" therapies. More recently approved drugs like abiraterone and enzalutamide are hormone-based treatments that are active in patients resistant to older therapies, hence the move from "hormone-refractory" to "castration-refractory" as the preferred terminology.

Prostate-specific antigen and hormone therapy

PSA is not recognized as a surrogate endpoint for clinical trials in relapsing disease when nonhormonal therapies are used [15]; however, early in hormone-sensitive disease, the concordance between PSA changes and clinical outcomes is close. One consequence of the use of the PSA test is that patients tend to have PSA- rather than clinically driven management. For patients relapsing after failed local therapy, clinicians are faced with a rising PSA but often no radiological evidence of disease for many years. This is called a biochemical relapse. Patients in this situation will often be started on hormone therapy many years before any clinical consequences of relapse are apparent. Results from randomized trials in this setting have shown that intermittent hormone therapy is as beneficial as continuous therapy [16]. Even more difficult for nonmetastatic patients is the next phase of castration-refractory biochemical relapse, which again may go on for years. Eventually, patients with biochemical relapse will develop radiological or clinical evidence of metastasis.

Once PSA levels start to rise, clinicians often try a second hormone manipulation, though the evidence to support this is scant. In particular, patients with metastatic disease and a rapidly rising PSA level run the risk of significant clinical problems if subjected to a trial of a second-line hormone therapy, so this practice is not recommended by the author. At the other end of the spectrum, patients with slowly rising PSA levels in the nonmetastatic setting often will undergo several courses of these second-line treatments; however, this may soon change due to advances in hormone therapies and imaging technologies. More recently, the use of steroids as a control arm in landmark trials with mitoxantrone [17] and abiraterone [18,19] has provided useful data on response rates to these latter agents in metastatic disease, both in first- and second-line settings.

Currently available hormone therapies

Gonadotropin-releasing hormone agonists

The gonadotropin-releasing hormone (GnRH) agonists were initially developed in the 1980s and have formed the mainstay of therapy for advanced prostate cancer for over 30 years. They act by binding to the pituitary gonadotropins as "super-agonists," resulting in an initial rise in the levels of luteinizing hormone and follicle-stimulating hormone, followed by an exhaustion of the cellular response and a fall to low levels of these hormones by 3–4 weeks of therapy. The testicular response mirrors this with an initial rise in testosterone followed by a fall to castration levels [20]. To block the stimulatory effects this might have on the cancer, termed "tumor flare," initiation of GnRH agonist therapy must be accompanied by an oral anti-androgen. Initial treatments were nasal sprays, but now all come in depot preparations of durations that vary from one month to one year.

Gonadotropin-releasing hormone receptor antagonists

In an attempt to avoid the risk of tumor flare, attempts have been made to develop pure GnRH receptor antagonists. Only one such preparation, degarelix, is marketed in the UK and is also available in the USA. Antagonists provide more rapid and more complete suppression of testosterone than the agonists, but currently are only available as monthly preparations, compared with the agonists where depot durations of up to a year can be obtained. The more rapid and complete testosterone suppression is potentially an advantage where disease burden is high and risks of complications, such as spinal cord compression, exist, or where compliance with oral anti-androgen therapy is considered problematic.

Figure 3.5 shows the relative effects of a GnRH agonist and antagonist on testosterone levels [21].

Hormone therapy for castration-resistant prostate cancer

Research has elucidated the mechanisms responsible for resistance to hormone therapy, and two themes emerge [22]:

- Changes in intraprostatic androgen synthesis:
  - Increased expression of enzymes converting dehydroepiandrosterone to testosterone and dihydrotestosterone in tumor tissue
  - Increased androgen synthesis
- Androgen receptor (AR) abnormalities:
  - Increased AR expression
  - Mutation of the AR ligand binding domain
  - Constitutively active AR mutants (truncated AR)

As these factors came to be better understood, it was possible to select new drug targets for development. The first agent to complete the development cycle was abiraterone, a drug initially synthesized in 1990. Abiraterone acts

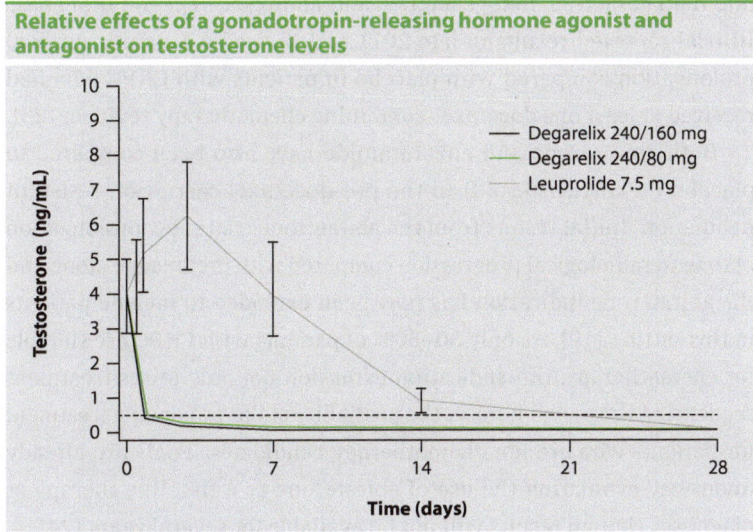

Figure 3.5 Relative effects of a gonadotropin-releasing hormone agonist and antagonist on testosterone levels. Reproduced with permission from © John Wiley and Sons, Klotz et al, 2013 [21]. All rights reserved.

by inhibiting the activities of the CYP17 enzyme, which promotes androgen biosynthesis. By interfering with androgen biosynthesis and thus the production of androgen, abiraterone decreases the level of androgen available to trigger the androgen receptor. A pivotal Phase III trial recruited patients with metastatic CRPC who had received docetaxel chemotherapy and randomized them to receive either abiraterone plus prednisone or placebo plus prednisone [18]. Treatment with abiraterone led to a 35% reduction in the risk of death compared with placebo. Patients taking abiraterone also had a better PSA response rate than patients taking placebo, and a 42% reduction in the risk of disease progression. The number of adverse events was similar between the two groups; the most common adverse events were fatigue, back pain, constipation, bone pain, and arthralgia [18]. The trial was stopped early by the Data Monitoring Committee, as it was considered unethical to leave patients on placebo.

A second compound, enzalutamide, is an AR antagonist with around a five-fold greater affinity for the receptor than bicalutamide. In addition, enzalutamide inhibits both nuclear translocation of the ligand:AR complex and androgen receptor-mediated DNA binding, a property that differentiates it from first-generation anti-androgens. The AFFIRM Phase III trial reported results in late 2011 and showed a 5-month survival prolongation compared with placebo in patients with CRPC who had received at least one docetaxel-containing chemotherapy regimen [23].

Both abiraterone and enzalutamide have also been compared to placebo (± corticosteroid) in the pre-docetaxel castration-resistant population. Initial results from the abiraterone trial show prolongation of time to radiological progression compared with prednisone alone and the abiraterone indication has now been extended to include patients in this setting [19]. As only 30–50% of patients with CRPC are suitable for chemotherapy, this indication extension not only raises treatment sequencing issues, but it raises the possibility of life-prolonging treatment for patients who are not chemotherapy candidates. Trials are already underway evaluating the use of abiraterone as a first-line therapy at diagnosis, though results will not be available for several years [24].

Preliminary results from the Phase III PREVAIL pre-chemotherapy study indicated that a statistically significant survival advantage was seen with enzalutamide treatment versus placebo ($p<0.0001$) in patients with metastatic prostate cancer who progressed despite ADT. Enzalutamide therapy led to a 30% reduction in the risk of death and an 81% reduction in the risk of radiographic progression or death. Based on the favorable benefit–risk ratio that enzalutamide demonstrated, the Independent Data Monitoring Committee recommended that the trial be stopped and patients receiving placebo be offered enzalutamide [25].

Sipuleucel-T has been recently approved in Europe for patients with asymptomatic or minimally symptomatic metastatic CRPC. The approval was based primarily on the Phase III IMPACT study [26] (n=512), which reported an improvement in overall survival compared to control (median survival varied from 2.8–13 months from lowest to highest PSA quartiles, respectively).

Emerging therapies for castration-resistant prostate cancer

Over the last few years, a number of therapies have entered trials for CRPC, two of which, abiraterone and enzalutamide, are now approved, with data pending on additional agents (see Table 3.3) [18,23,26–30].

Trials for castration-resistant prostate cancer				
Trial (year); agent	Setting	Control arm	Hazard ratio	p value
IMPACT (2010) [26]; sipuleucel-T	Chemo-naïve CRPC	Placebo	0.775	0.032
Tax327 (2004) [27]; docetaxel	Chemo-naïve CRPC	Mitoxantrone	0.76	0.09
TROPIC (2010) [28]; cabazitaxel	Post-docetaxel CRPC	Mitoxantrone	0.70	<0.0001
COU-AA-301 (2011) [18]; abiraterone	Post-docetaxel CRPC	Placebo	0.646	<0.0001
ALSYMPCA (2012) [29,30]; radium-223	Pre- or post-chemotherapy CRPC	Placebo	0.695	0.00185
AFFIRM (2012) [23]; enzalutamide	Post-docetaxel CRPC	Placebo	0.63	<0.001

Table 3.3 Trials for castration-resistant prostate cancer. CRPC, castration-resistant prostate cancer. de Bono et al [18], Scher et al [23], Kantoff et al [26], Tannock et al [27], de Bono et al [28], Brady et al [29], Parker et al [30].

Combining hormone therapy with radiotherapy

Landmark trials have demonstrated conclusively that adding hormone therapy to radiotherapy improved outcomes for patients with locally advanced disease, including overall survival [31]. Moreover, a short-term course (4–6 months) of hormone therapy and radiotherapy appeared sufficient to confer most of the observed benefit. RTOG 8610 compared 4 months of hormone therapy plus radiotherapy (to 65–70 Gy) with radiotherapy alone, and showed clear improvements in disease-free, metastasis-free, and overall survival, sustained for at least 15 years post-treatment [31].

Other studies have examined longer durations of hormone therapy. The EORTC 22863 trial compared radiotherapy alone with radiotherapy plus 3 years of hormone therapy, with 5-year survival rates improving from 62% to 79% [32]. Other studies suggested that the bulk of the benefit from the longer duration of therapy is in patients with the highest-risk disease (higher PSA values, Gleason scores 8–10, or T3–4 disease) [33].

Studies comparing hormone therapy alone or hormone therapy plus radiotherapy were initiated to determine whether radiotherapy was unnecessary due to the striking survival benefit observed with short durations of hormone therapy. Data from two large studies, SPCG-7 [34] and PR07 [35], showed the unequivocal benefit of combination therapy. Results from SPCG-7 are illustrated in Figure 3.6 [34].

With improving technology, radiation doses have gradually escalated, based on the assumption that reduced normal tissue damage would allow the dose to be increased, improving outcomes. However, a survival advantage has not been established with dose escalation. For example, the RT01 trial compared short term hormone therapy plus radiotherapy (to either 64 Gy or 74 Gy) and noted a substantial improvement in 5-year PSA relapse rates [36]. Yet, longer-term follow-up has failed to show any benefit in overall survival and, more surprisingly, in metastasis-free survival as well. There is thus little to justify escalation beyond 74 Gy in 2-Gy fractions. More recently, there has been much interest in treating patients with shorter courses at larger doses per fraction, based on radiobiological observations, suggesting an improved therapeutic ratio

Hormone therapy versus hormone therapy plus radiotherapy from SPCG-7 study

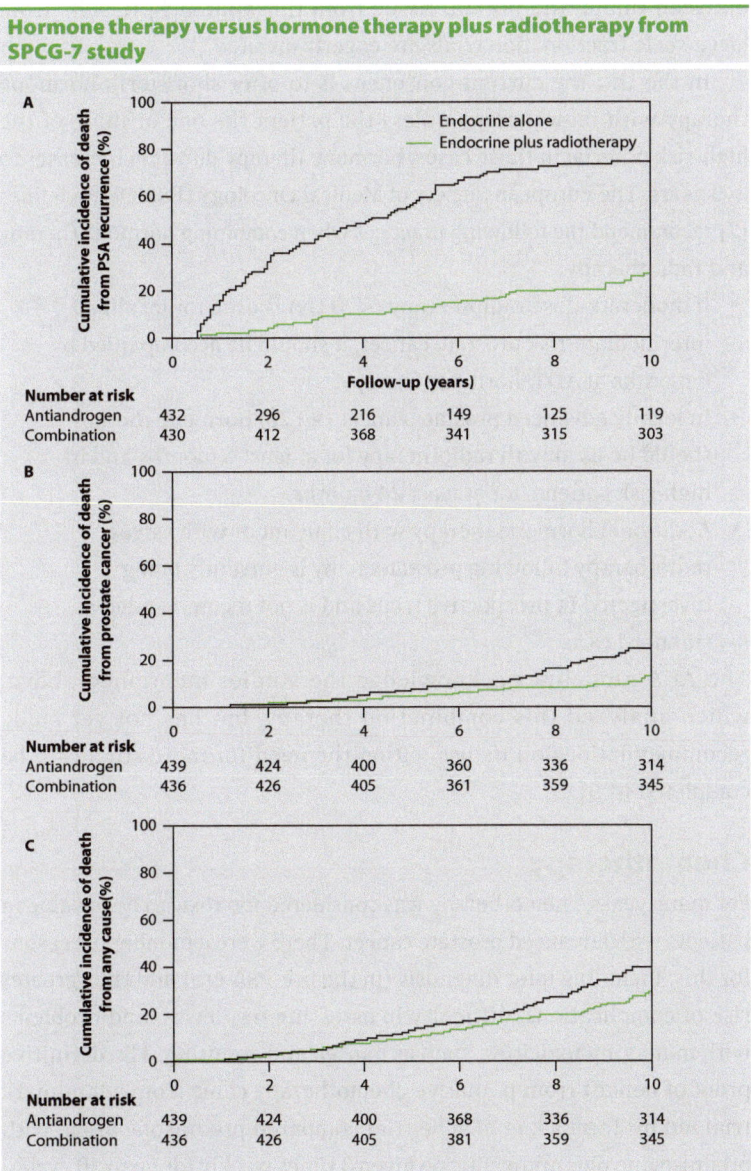

Figure 3.6 Hormone therapy versus hormone therapy plus radiotherapy from SPCG-7 study. A, PSA relapse-free survival; B, disease-specific survival; C, overall survival. PSA, prostate-specific antigen. Reproduced with permission © Lancet, Widmark et al, 2013 [34]. All Rights Reserved.

between tumor and normal tissue from this approach. Results from large-scale fractionation trials are eagerly awaited.

In the UK, the current consensus is to offer short-term hormone therapy with radiotherapy unless the patient fits one or more of the high-risk criteria; in those cases, hormone therapy duration increases to 2–3 years. The European Society of Medical Oncology (ESMO) guidelines [2] recommend the following practices when combining hormone therapy and radiotherapy:

- If moderate-dose radiotherapy (<70 Gy) is used for localized intermediate-risk prostate cancer, it should be accompanied by 6 months of ADT/hormone therapy.
- In locally advanced prostate cancer (≥T2b) hormone therapy should be used with radiotherapy for at least 6 months and in high-risk patients for at least 24 months.
- Additional hormone therapy with adjuvant or with salvage radiotherapy following prostatectomy is currently being investigated in prospective trials and is not recommended as standard care.

The AUA guidelines acknowledge the studies mentioned above, which analyzed this combination therapy, but has not yet made recommendations on its use, citing the need for more studies to be completed [4,5].

Chemotherapy

For many years, chemotherapy was considered too toxic to be of value in patients with advanced prostate cancer. There were a number of reasons for this, including later diagnosis (in the pre-PSA era) and thus greater risk of complications, difficulty in assessing responses, and problems with managing toxicities, such as nausea and vomiting. The definitive proof of benefit from palliative chemotherapy came from a landmark trial led by Tannock et al. The trial compared prednisone alone with prednisolone plus mitoxantrone given 3 times weekly for up to 10 cycles. This relatively small study of 161 patients published in 1996 set out to compare palliative endpoints rather than survival-based ones [17]. A palliative response was observed in 28.8% of patients who received mitoxantrone plus prednisone, compared with 12.3% of patients who received prednisone alone. An additional seven patients in each group reduced their analgesic medication without an increase in pain [17]. The duration of palliation was longer in patients who received chemotherapy, with a median of 43 weeks to symptom worsening with chemotherapy compared to 18 weeks with prednisone alone. There was significant crossover from the prednisone arm to chemotherapy and no difference in overall survival. This study thus clearly established the principle that chemotherapy could provide palliative benefit, but did not show a survival benefit [17]. Subsequent mitoxantrone trials produced similar results [37,38], though the crossover between the chemotherapy and no-chemotherapy arms means it is essentially unknown if chemotherapy with this agent produces a survival benefit or not.

Docetaxel

In the late 1990s, a variety of agents started to be evaluated for patients with CRPC. Docetaxel emerged as the lead candidate for evaluation in large-phase trials and two landmark studies were published in the *New England Journal of Medicine* in 2004. One trial, the TAX327 study, compared weekly or three-times weekly docetaxel with the Tannock mitoxantrone regimen [27]. The second trial (SWOG 9916) compared a combination of docetaxel and estramustine with the same control arm [39]. Both trials showed improved palliative outcomes versus mitoxantrone, and most importantly an overall survival advantage for three-times weekly docetaxel and the docetaxel-estramustine combination, with hazard ratios of 0.76 and 0.8 respectively, despite significant crossover to docetaxel in the mitoxantrone arms of both studies [27,39]. All patients in both trials received prednisone as per the original Tannock paper. These trials confirmed that chemotherapy could both prolong survival and give palliation without undue toxicity. They also established that docetaxel was a superior agent to mitoxantrone [27,39]. On the basis of simplicity and toxicity, the three times weekly docetaxel plus prednisone regimen became established as the standard of care in metastatic CRPC.

The post-docetaxel era

Subsequent research has focused on a number of areas: earlier use of docetaxel, use of docetaxel in combination with other agents, and development of new chemotherapy drugs for second-line therapy. In numerous combination-therapy trials, no study combination with optimally delivered docetaxel has shown a significant improvement compared with docetaxel alone, which thus remains the standard of care. Two large trials, GETUG-15 and STAMPEDE, have found that upfront docetaxel prolongs time to progression. The GETUG-15 data have recently been presented and note an improved time to progression, with a hazard ratio of 0.72–0.75, but no improvement in overall survival [40]. The STAMPEDE trial is somewhat larger, and an interim (unpublished) analysis confirms an improvement in failure-free survival sufficient to continue the trial to completion (note: the trial met the published criteria in the statistics plan to complete recruitment). Initial survival data from STAMPEDE are expected in 2015.

A number of chemotherapy agents have been studied in the second-line setting. Currently, only cabazitaxel has shown a survival advantage and obtained approval. The key trial, TROPIC, compared cabazitaxel with mitoxantrone given on the standard Tannock trial schedule and showed an improvement in median survival from 12.7 to 15.1 months. The overall survival data from TROPIC are given in Figure 3.7 [28].

Bone-targeting therapies

Metastases from prostate cancer commonly occur in the lymph nodes, lungs, liver, adrenal gland, and brain; however, when prostate cancer becomes metastatic, it almost always progresses to the bones [41,42].

The actual prevalence of bone metastases varies with duration of relapse and pattern of disease at presentation [27,39]. There are a growing number of therapies available to target bone metastasis, both for treating symptoms and also for preventing bone complications, such as spinal cord compression, pain, and fracture. In recent literature, the impact of bone-targeting therapies has been assessed with a composite measure termed the skeletal-related event (SRE). The elements that make up this endpoint are:

- pathological fracture,
- spinal cord compression,
- radiotherapy to bone,
- hypocalcemia, and
- change in anti-cancer treatment to treat bone pain.

These elements vary in clinical significance and are also, to a degree, subjective. In particular, the zoledronic acid [43] and more recent denosumab [44] approval trials have proved very controversial, as the fracture endpoint was assessed by regular skeletal survey with blinded radiological assessment. Hence, there is significant doubt as to whether many of the small fractures detected were precursors of a subsequent real "clinical" SRE or radiological features of no significance. The subsequent trials comparing zoledronic acid with denosumab [44] used the same

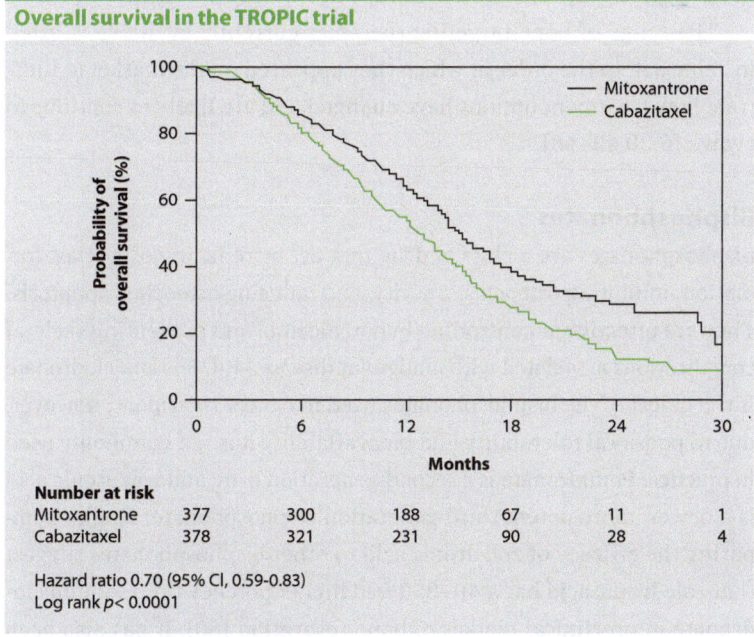

Overall survival in the TROPIC trial

Number at risk

Mitoxantrone	377	300	188	67	11	1
Cabazitaxel	378	321	231	90	28	4

Hazard ratio 0.70 (95% CI, 0.59-0.83)
Log rank $p < 0.0001$

Figure 3.7 Overall survival in the TROPIC trial. Compares cabazitaxel with mitoxantrone in patients previously treated with docetaxel. Reproduced with permission from © Lancet, de Bono et al, 2013 [28]. All Rights Reserved.

methodology and can, therefore, be subject to the same criticism. As a result, neither agent is recommended for the prevention of SREs in patients with metastatic prostate cancer in the UK by the National Institute of Health and Care Excellence (NICE), though in the opinion of the author, prevention of bone complications with relatively low-toxicity therapies is better than managing the complications when they arise. Both agents are approved in the USA and EU, specifically denosumab is approved for the prevention of SREs in patients with bone metastases from solid tumors and zoledronic acid is approved for patients with documented bone metastases from prostate cancer who have progressed after treatment with at least one hormonal therapy.

In contrast, the radium-223 licensing trial ALSYMPCA used overall survival as the primary endpoint, with clinical SRE as a secondary endpoint. The trial was positive for a survival advantage, and showed a highly significant reduction in clinical SREs [30]. The agent received approval in the USA in May 2013 and in Europe in November 2013.

The range of bone-targeting therapies currently available is listed in Table 3.4, in the order in which they appeared on the market to illustrate how treatment options have changed and are likely to continue to evolve [6,30,43–48].

Bisphosphonates

Bisphosphonates are a class of drug that act by reducing osteoclast formation, inhibiting osteoclast activity, and inducing osteoclast apoptosis. They are effective at controlling hypercalcemia and preventing skeletal complications associated with malignant disease [49]. Sodium clodronate is the oldest of the bisphosphonates used in cancer treatment; however, due to poor oral tolerability and bioavailability it is not commonly used in practice. Pamidronate is a second-generation drug and zoledronic acid is a newer, more potent third-generation bisphosphonate; studies comparing the efficacy of zoledronic acid to other bisphosphonates suggest that zoledronic acid has a 40–850 fold higher potency than sodium clodronate in preclinical models of bone resorption [50]. It has also been shown to be more effective than pamidronate in controlling malignant hypercalcemia [51]. Furthermore, trials have shown a lack of efficacy for

Bone-targeting therapies

Treatment	Indications	Limitations
Palliative radiotherapy [6]	Bone pain	Loss of bone marrow function, retreatments limited
Strontium-89 [45]	Bone pain	Myelosuppression
Samarium-153 lexidronam [46]	Bone pain	Myelosuppression
Sodium clodronate [47]	Bone pain	Gastrointestinal toxicity, limited efficacy
Zoledronic acid [30,43]	Bone pain, prevention of SRE	Nephrotoxicity, regular intravenous treatments needed, risk of osteonecrosis of jaw
Denosumab [44,48]	Prevention of SRE (pathological fracture, radiation to bone, spinal cord compression or surgery to bone) in adults with bone metastases from solid tumors	Regular subcutaneous injections needed, risk of osteonecrosis of jaw
Alendronate [48]	Postmenopausal osteoporosis in patients at risk of vitamin D insufficiency; reduces the risk of vertebral and hip fractures	May cause upper gastrointestinal adverse events, osteonecrosis of jaw, musculoskeletal pain, atypical fractures of the femur, renal insufficiency, issues with bone and mineral metabolism, and hypercalcemia or hypercalciuria
Radium Ra 223 dichloride [30]	Treatment for patients with CRPC, symptomatic bone metastases, and no known visceral metastatic disease	Myelosuppression, repeated intravenous injections, more complicated radiation protection than strontium-89 and samarium-153 lexidronam

Table 3.4 Bone-targeting therapies. CRPC, castration-resistant prostate cancer; SRE, skeletal-related event. Adapted from Cookson et al [6], Parker et al [30], Saad et al [43], Fizazi et al [44], Porter and McEwan [45], Sartor et al [46], Dearnaley et al [47], National Comprehensive Cancer Center [48].

pamidronate as well in preventing bone events [52]. Data suggest that the early use of bisphosphonates in metastatic bone disease may improve survival [47]. Zoledronic acid has the most convincing evidence base, with a substantial delay in time to first SRE and reduction in subsequent SRE numbers compared with placebo (Figure 3.8) [43].

Several trials have investigated the use of zoledronic acid in the preventative setting by introducing bone protection at the time of diagnosis. These include STAMPEDE and the European ZEUS trial. Results from both studies are expected in the coming years. Until data become

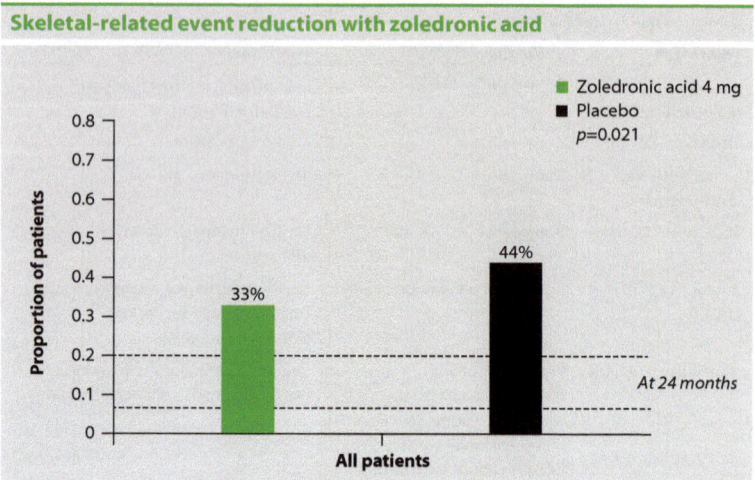

Figure 3.8 Skeletal-related event reduction with zoledronic acid. Adapted from Saad et al [43].

available, this author recommends that the use of zoledronic acid should be restricted to patients with CRPC [43].

Denosumab

Denosumab is a monoclonal antibody that targets the RANK ligand, an element in the pathway that drives bone destruction via osteoclasts. Denosumab is not nephrotoxic and is given subcutaneously, so administration can be quick and less likely to be stopped for toxicity. The drug has been compared head-to-head with zoledronic acid in a Phase III study and was found to be more efficacious in terms of SRE prevention in patients with metastatic CRPC (Figure 3.9) [44]. Denosumab prolonged the median time to first on-study SRE by 3.6 months as compared with zoledronic acid. Overall survival (an exploratory endpoint) was similar between the denosumab and zoledronic acid groups. The safety profiles were also similar.

However, denosumab has been the focus of some controversy because its major trials used SREs as the primary endpoint; it also is not recommended by NICE, but is approved in the USA and EU.

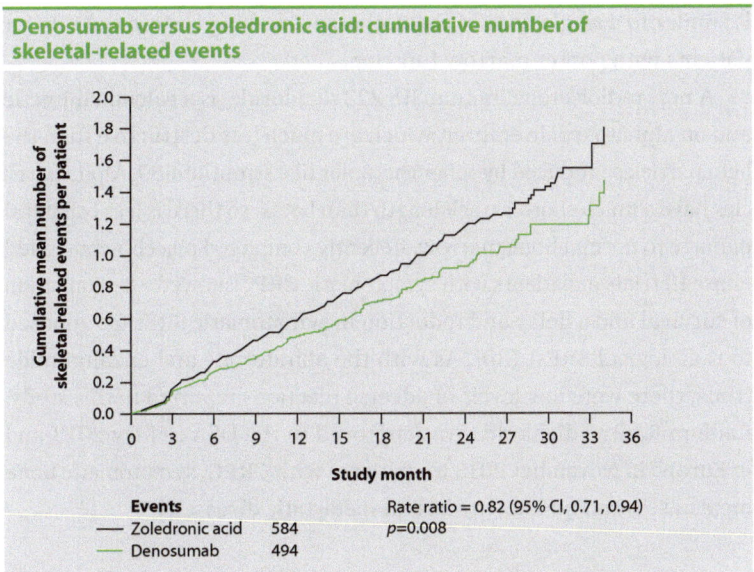

Figure 3.9 Denosumab versus zoledronic acid: cumulative number of skeletal-related events. Events occurring at least 21 days apart. Reproduced with permission from © Elsevier, Fizazi et al, 2013 [44]. All Rights Reserved.

Radioisotopes

Radioisotope therapy with the isotope strontium-89 has been shown in pivotal trials to improve symptom control and reduce the need for further treatments, such as radiotherapy [45]. Its mode of action depends on strontium being a calcium mimetic and it is therefore incorporated at high concentrations in the osteoblastic reaction associated with prostate cancer bone metastasis. The agent has both a long physical half-life and long persistence in bone cells due to this incorporation effect. This gives a long duration of pain relief – often over 3 months – but also a risk of damage to normal bone marrow, with consequent bone marrow failure in some cases.

Samarium-153 lexidronam is approved for the relief of pain in patients with confirmed osteoblastic metastatic bone lesions that enhance on a radionuclide bone scan [53,54]. Samarium-153 lexidronam has a short half-life, so although it is myelotoxic, the duration of marrow suppression is similar to a single dose of chemotherapy, making it more suitable for patients with poorer marrow function.

A new radioisotope, radium Ra 223 dichloride, is a calcium mimetic and an alpha-particle emitter, which are much less destructive than the beta particles produced by other therapies like strontium-89. Alpha particles have a much shorter track length than betas, so there is less collateral damage to normal bone marrow. Recently completed placebo-controlled Phase III trials in patients with symptomatic CRPC showed a prolongation of survival and a delay and reduction in symptomatic SREs (as opposed to radiological SREs) [30]. As with the abiraterone and enzalutamide trials, there were low levels of adverse reactions reported in this study. Radium Ra 223 dichloride was approved in the USA in May 2013 and in Europe in November 2013 for patients with CRPC, symptomatic bone metastases, and no known visceral metastatic disease.

Summary

Treatment options for prostate cancer are not homogenous across the risk spectrum. For low-risk patients, active monitoring is increasingly seen as the treatment of choice, especially in patients with significant comorbidities [55]. As the aggressiveness of the tumor intensifies, the risk of harm from untreated cancer also grows, increasing the need for treatment. The Scandinavian SPCG-4 trial comparing prostatectomy with watchful waiting identified patients with extra-capsular spread as benefiting most from surgery [56]. For low- to intermediate-risk cancers, locally ablative techniques (surgery, brachytherapy, and HIFU or cryotherapy) are appropriate. As the risk of local spread and capsular involvement increases, these treatments become less attractive due to greater potential for untreated disease at the margins. For intermediate- to high-risk cases, the need for systemic therapy to treat possible micrometastatic spread rises. Based on this author's clinical experience, this is best combined with radiotherapy and both treatments are needed for tumor control and to reduce the risk of death. As we move to higher-risk cases, it seems increasingly unjustified to subject patients to surgery when both local spread and distant disease can be addressed with lower morbidity with combinations of hormone therapy and radiotherapy.

References

1   Heidenreich A, Bellmunt J, Bolla M, et al. EAU guidelines on prostate cancer. Part I: screening, diagnosis, and treatment of clinically localised disease. *Eur Urol*. 2011;59:61-71.

2   Mottet N, Bellmunt J, Bolla M, et al. EAU guidelines on prostate cancer. Part II: treatment of advanced, relapsing, and castration-resistant prostate cancer. *Eur Urol*. 2011;59:572-583.

3   Horwich A, Hugosson J, de Reijke T, Wiegel T, Fizazi K, Kataja V; Panel Members. Prostate cancer: ESMO Consensus Conference guidelines 2012. *Ann Oncol*. 2013;24:1141-1162.

4   American Urological Association. Guideline for the management of clinically localized prostate cancer: 2007 update. www.auanet.org/common/pdf/education/clinical-guidance/Prostate-Cancer.pdf. Accessed July 18, 2013.

5   Thompson IM , Valicenti R, Albertsen PC, et al. Adjuvant and salvage radiotherapy after prostatectomy: ASTRO/AUA guideline. www.auanet.org/common/pdf/education/clinical-guidance/Radiation-After-Prostatectomy.pdf. Accessed July 18, 2013.

6   Cookson MS, Roth BJ, Dahm P, et al. Castration-resistant prostate cancer: AUA guideline. *J Urol*. 2013;190:429-438.

7   Walsh PC, Lepor H. The role of radical prostatectomy in the management of prostatic cancer. *Cancer*. 1997;60(3 suppl):526-537.

8   Finkelstein J, Eckersberger E, Sadri H, Taneja SS, Lepor H, Djavan B. Open versus laparoscopic versus robot-assisted laparoscopic prostatectomy: the European and US experience. *Rev Urol*. 2010;12:35-43.

9   Heidenreich A, Varga Z, Von Knobloch R. Extended pelvic lymphadenectomy in patients undergoing radical prostatectomy: high incidence of lymph node metastasis. *J Urol*. 2002;167:1681-1686.

10 Mayo Clinic. Cryotherapy for prostate cancer. Risks. www.mayoclinic.com/health/cryotherapy-for-prostate-cancer/MY01634/DSECTION=risks. Accessed July 18, 2013.

11 Pommier P, Chabaud S, Lagrange JL, et al. Is there a role for pelvic irradiation in localized prostate adenocarcinoma? Preliminary results of GETUG-01. *J Clin Oncol*. 2007;25:5366-5373.

12 Theodorescu D. Prostate cancer, clinical oncology. In: Schwab M, ed. *Encyclopedic Reference of Cancer*. Berlin, Germany: Springer-Verlag; 2001:720-727.

13 CyberKnife. Side Effects: Prostate. www.cyberknife.com/Content.aspx?id=5404. Accessed July 18, 2013.

14 Huggins C, Hodges CV. Studies on prostatic cancer. I. The effect of castration, of estrogen and androgen injection on serum phosphatases in metastatic carcinoma of the prostate. *Cancer Res*. 1941;1:293-297.

15 Bubley GJ, Carducci M, Dahut W, et al. Eligibility and response guidelines for phase II clinical trials in androgen-independent prostate cancer: recommendations from the Prostate-Specific Antigen Working Group. *J Clin Oncol*. 1999;17:3461-3467.

16 Crook JM, O'Callaghan CJ, Duncan G, et al. Intermittent androgen suppression for rising PSA level after radiotherapy. *N Engl J Med*. 2012;367:895-903.

17 Tannock IF, Osoba D, Stockler MR, et al. Chemotherapy with mitoxantrone plus prednisone or prednisone alone for symptomatic hormone-resistant prostate cancer: a Canadian randomized trial with palliative end points. *J Clin Oncol*. 1996;14:1756-1764.

18 de Bono JS, Logothetis CJ, Molina A, et al; for the COU-AA-301 Investigators. Abiraterone and increased survival in metastatic prostate cancer. *N Engl J Med*. 2011;364:1995-2005.

19 Ryan CJ, Smith MR, de Bono JS, et al; for the COU-AA-302 Investigators. Abiraterone in metastatic prostate cancer without previous chemotherapy. *N Engl J Med*. 2013;368:138-148.

20 Trachtenberg J, Gittleman M, Steidle C, et al; Abarelix Study Group. A phase 3, multicenter, open label, randomized study of abarelix versus leuprolide plus daily antiandrogen in men with prostate cancer. *J Urol*. 2002;167:1670-1674.

21 Klotz L, Boccon-Gibod L, Shore ND, et al. The efficacy and safety of degarelix: a 12-month, comparative, randomized, open-label, parallel-group phase III study in patients with prostate cancer. *BJU Int*. 2008;102:1531-1538.

22 Labrie F. Blockade of testicular and adrenal androgens in prostate cancer treatment. *Nat Rev Urol*. 2011;8:73-85.

23 Scher HI, Fizazi K, Saad F, et al; for the AFFIRM Investigators. Increased survival with enzalutamide in prostate cancer after chemotherapy. *N Engl J Med*. 2012;367:1187-1197.

24 Sydes MR, James ND, Mason MD, et al. Flexible trial design in practice - dropping and adding arms in STAMPEDE: a multi-arm multi-stage randomised controlled trial. *Trials*. 2011;12(suppl 1):A3.

25 Medivation and Astellas announce the Phase 3 PREVAIL trial of enzalutamide meets both co-primary endpoints of overall survival and radiographic progression-free survival in chemotherapy-naive patients with advanced prostate cancer [press release October 22, 2013]. http://investors.medivation.com/releasedetail.cfm?ReleaseID=798880. Accessed October 24, 2013.

26 Kantoff PW, Higano CS, Shore ND, et al; for the IMPACT Study Investigators. Sipuleucel-T immunotherapy for castration-resistant prostate cancer. *N Engl J Med*. 2010;363:411-422.

27 Tannock IF, de Wit R, Berry WR, et al; for the TAX 327 Investigators. Docetaxel plus prednisone or mitoxantrone plus prednisone for advanced prostate cancer. *N Engl J Med*. 2004;351:1502-1512.

28 de Bono JS, Oudard S, Ozguroglu M, et al; for the TROPIC Investigators. Prednisone plus cabazitaxel or mitoxantrone for metastatic castration-resistant prostate cancer progressing after docetaxel treatment: a randomised open-label trial. *Lancet*. 2010;376:1147-1154.

29 Brady D, Parker CC, O'Sullivan JM. Bone-targeting radiopharmaceuticals including radium-223. *Cancer J*. 2013;19:71-78.

30 Parker C, Nilsson S, Heinrich D, et al. Alpha emitter radium-223 and survival in metastatic prostate cancer. *N Engl J Med*. 2013;369:213-223.

31 Roach M III, Bae K, Speight J, et al. Short-term neoadjuvant androgen deprivation therapy and external-beam radiotherapy for locally advanced prostate cancer: long-term results of RTOG 8610. *J Clin Oncol*. 2008;26:585-591.

32 Bolla M, Van Tienhoven G, Warde P, et al. External irradiation with or without long-term androgen suppression for prostate cancer with high metastatic risk: 10-year results of an EORTC randomized study. *Lancet Oncol*. 2010;11:1066-1073.

33 Pilepich MV, Caplan R, Byhardt RW, et al. Phase III trial of androgen suppression using goserelin in unfavorable-prognosis carcinoma of the prostate treated with definitive radiotherapy: report of Radiation Therapy Oncology Group Protocol 85-31. *J Clin Oncol*. 1997;15:1013-1021.

34 Widmark A, Klepp O, Solberg A, et al; for the Scandinavian Prostate Cancer Group Study 7/ the Swedish Association for Urological Oncology 3. Endocrine treatment, with or without radiotherapy, in locally advanced prostate cancer (SPCG-7/SFUO-3): an open randomised phase III trial. *Lancet*. 2009;373:301-308.

35 Warde P, Mason M, Ding K, et al; for the NCIC CTG PR.3/MRC UK PR07 Investigators. Combined androgen deprivation therapy and radiation therapy for locally advanced prostate cancer: a randomised, phase 3 trial. *Lancet*. 2011;378:2104-2111.

36 Dearnaley DP, Sydes MR, Graham JD, et al; on behalf of the RT01 Collaborators. Escalated-dose versus standard-dose conformal radiotherapy in prostate cancer: first results from the MRC RT01 randomised controlled trial. *Lancet Oncol*. 2007;8:475-487.

37 Kantoff PW, Halabi S, Conaway M, et al. Hydrocortisone with or without mitoxantrone in men with hormone-refractory prostate cancer: results of the Cancer and Leukemia Group B 9182 study. *J Clin Oncol*. 1999;17:2506-2513.

38 Berry W, Dakhil S, Modiano M, Gregurich M, Asmar L. Phase III study of mitoxantrone plus low dose prednisone versus low dose prednisone alone in patients with asymptomatic hormone refractory prostate cancer. *J Urol*. 2002;168:2439-2443.

39 Petrylak DP, Tangen CM, Hussain MHA, et al. Docetaxel and estramustine compared with mitoxantrone and prednisone for advanced refractory prostate cancer. *N Engl J Med*. 2004;351:1513-1520.

40 Gravis G, Fizazi K, Joly F, et al. Androgen-deprivation therapy alone or with docetaxel in non-castrate metastatic prostate cancer (GETUG-AFU 15): a randomised, open-label, phase 3 trial. *Lancet Oncol*. 2013;14:149-158.

41 Mayo Clinic. Prostate Cancer. www.mayoclinic.com/health/prostate-cancer-metastasis/AN02203. Accessed July 18, 2013.

42 National Cancer Institute. Metastatic Cancer. www.cancer.gov/cancertopics/factsheet/Sites-Types/metastatic. Accessed July 18, 2013.

43 Saad F, Gleason DM, Murray R, et al; for the Zoledronic Acid Prostate Cancer Study Group. Long-term efficacy of zoledronic acid for the prevention of skeletal complications in patients with metastatic hormone-refractory prostate cancer. *J Natl Cancer Inst*. 2004;96:879-882.

44 Fizazi K, Carducci M, Smith M, et al. Denosumab versus zoledronic acid for treatment of bone metastases in men with castration-resistant prostate cancer: a randomised, double-blind study. *Lancet*. 2011;377:813-822.

45 Porter AT, McEwan AJ. Strontium-89 as an adjuvant to external beam radiation improves pain relief and delays disease progression in advanced prostate cancer: results of a randomized controlled trial. *Semin Oncol*. 1993;20:38-43.

46 Sartor O, Reid RH, Hoskin PJ, et al; Quadramet 424Sm10/11 Study Group. Samarium-153-lexidronam complex for treatment of painful bone metastases in hormone-refractory prostate cancer. *Urology*. 2004;63:940-945.

47 Dearnaley DP, Mason MD, Parmar MKB, Sanders K, Sydes MR. Adjuvant therapy with oral sodium clodronate in locally advanced and metastatic prostate cancer: long-term overall survival results from the MRC PR04 and PR05 randomised controlled trials. *Lancet Oncol*. 2009;10:872-876.

48 National Comprehensive Cancer Center (NCCN). NCCN clinical practice guidelines in oncology (NCCN Guideline®): prostate cancer. www.nccn.org/professionals/physician_gls/pdf/prostate.pdf. Accessed July 18, 2013.

49 Riccardi A, Grasso D, Danova M. Bisphosphonates in oncology: physiopathologic bases and clinical activity. *Tumori*. 2003;89:223-236.

50 Green JR, Müller K, Jaeggi KA. Preclinical pharmacology of CGP 42'446, a new, potent, heterocyclic bisphosphonate compound. *J Bone Miner Res*. 1994;9:745-751.

51 Major P, Lortholary A, Hon J, et al. Zoledronic acid is superior to pamidronate in the treatment of hypercalcemia of malignancy: a pooled analysis of two randomized, controlled clinical trials. *J Clin Oncol*. 2001;19:558-567.

52 Small EJ, Smith MR, Seaman JJ, Petrone S, Kowalski MO. Combined analysis of two multicenter, randomized, placebo-controlled studies of pamidronate disodium for the palliation of bone pain in men with metastatic prostate cancer. *J Clin Oncol*. 2003;21:4277-4284.

53 Serafini AN. Samarium Sm-153 lexidronam for the palliation of bone pain associated with metastases. *Cancer*. 2000;88(12 suppl):2934-2939.

54 QUADRAMET® [package insert]. Langhorne, PA: EUSA Pharma (USA), Inc; 2009.

55 Wilt TJ, Brawer MK, Jones KM, et al; for the Prostate Cancer Intervention versus Observation Trial (PIVOT) Study Group. Radical prostatectomy versus observation for localized prostate cancer. *N Engl J Med*. 2012;367:203-213.

56 Bill-Axelson A, Holmberg L, Ruutu M, et al; for the SPCG-4 Investigators. Radical prostatectomy versus watchful waiting in early prostate cancer. *N Engl J Med*. 2011;364:1708-1717.

Chapter 4

Conclusions

Management for patients with prostate cancer is quickly evolving. At one end of the spectrum, there is a growing realization that early disease does not always need treating and that monitoring may be a reasonable option for many patients diagnosed with early prostate cancer. For those who require treatment, the range of options continues to grow, with less-invasive surgical, quasi-surgical techniques, and improved radiotherapy technologies becoming available.

At the other end of the spectrum, the options for those with relapsed disease continue to change and are summarized in Figure 4.1. New drugs with distinct modes of action have been approved in recent years, with the promise of further new agents to come. Radium Ra 223 dichloride has been approved in the USA for relapsing metastatic disease, and was approved in Europe in November 2013. Thus, three agents will be available in the USA and EU as first-line therapies in patients with relapsing metastatic

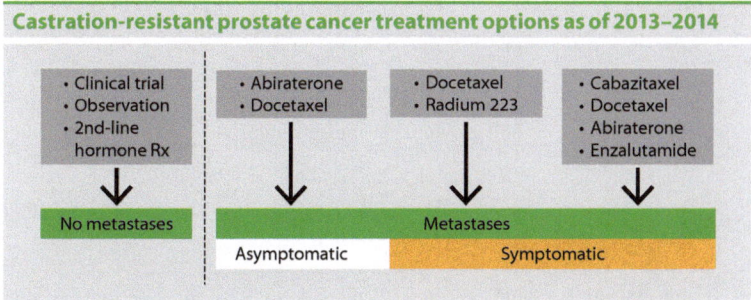

Figure 4.1 Castration-resistant prostate cancer treatment options as of 2013–2014.

N. James, *Primer on Prostate Cancer*,
DOI: 10.1007/978-1-907673-82-5_4, © Springer Healthcare 2014

disease—docetaxel, abiraterone, and radium Ra 223 dichloride—with enzalutamide possibly set to join the list when the pre-chemotherapy trial matures, as well as the possibility additional agents to come. Unraveling how to use these emerging therapeutic options will be a challenge for both professionals conducting clinical trials and managing patients with prostate cancer for many years to come.